Endomorph Diet Guide Made Quite Simple:

Reliable Secrets & Approaches to Burning up Fats as an Endomorph Speedily; Inclusion of the Right Meal Plan for You & the Required Exercises

By

Dr. Annette B. Eichel
Copyright@2021

TABLE OF CONTENTS

THE END...36

CHAPTER 1

INTRODUCTION

It is totally a priceless, basic notwithstanding practice plan for a social affair folks that are in the endomorph kind of body, and who are doing and combating to snatch hold or direct body weight, and generally thriving.

It is fundamentally the suppers, sustenance or diets that are exclusively made for

the get-together of people
having more noteworthy
boned, having the opportunity
of getting more weight than
required.

The guide reveals how you
can without a very remarkable
stretch loss the troubles of
being an endomorph,
notwithstanding other
unprecedented things you
remain to benefit. Discover
these extraordinary thoughts
in the following chapters!

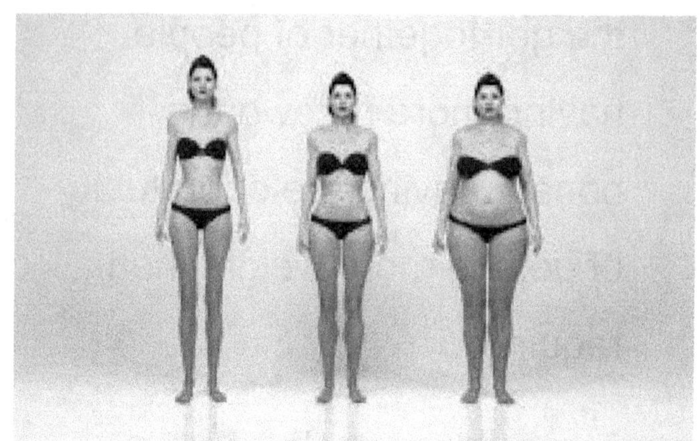

Ectomorph Mesomorph Endomorph

CHAPTER 2

DIET PLAN RECOMMENDED FOR ENDOMORPHS AS WELL AS THE MEALS TO BE INCLUDED IN THEIR DIET PLANS

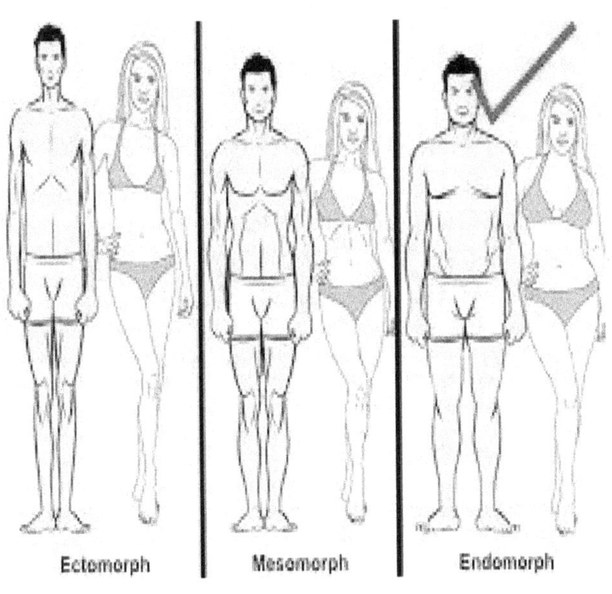

A Meal Plan Recommended for Endomorph Meals

Ideally, if you decide to improve your prosperity and follow an endomorph diet plan or decides that will manage you on the sorts or kinds of meals or food sources you should consume, notwithstanding the gathering of a sound lifestyle and a couple of changes in the time you eat up your dinners or food sources, you sure to experience inconceivable improvement. Likewise, this eating routine course of action includes long stretch organizing, and not actually a full scale departure of calorie; this eating routine arrangement makes one burn-through fat sufficiently and in a unique manner.

Plus, research reveals that the people who are endomorphs should go for avoids food that are contained the going with:

- 30% of starches

- 35 % of fat

- 35% of protein

Despite the previously mentioned, the fat make-up or creation should be satisfactory fats like grass-dealt with margarine, olive oil assembled spread (or ghee), avocado, etc What's more, for calorie decline confirmation for endomorphs, it should be between 340 to 500 for a common having routine or supper.

The Vital Foods or Meals to
Be Added in an Endomorph
Diet are Given Thus:

- Nuts

- Seeds

- Fatty fish

- Cheese having basically zero fat

- White chicken notwithstanding burger; lean protein

- Carbohydrates

- Protein powder

- Walnuts

- Beans and vegetables

- Healthy fats like olive oil

Further Imperative Things
You Should Know for an
Endomorph Meal

Here, the eating routine or banquet you need to make should have a mix of good or sound fats, protein notwithstanding vegetables.

Gain by Protein: Here, the usage of these food sources or dinners energizes one in muscles collecting, and doesn't store or keep fat in the body in at any rate.

Usage of plentiful Veggies: Now, the huge proportion of fiber notwithstanding its sustaining thickness weakens glutting and besides urges one to be involved on time.

Eating up Your Meals or Foods progressively: Here, you are asked to consume your dinners or sustenance continuously considering the way that it helps or encourages your body to know when you are really finished off.

CHAPTER3

THE BODY TYPES FREQUENTLY OBSERVED

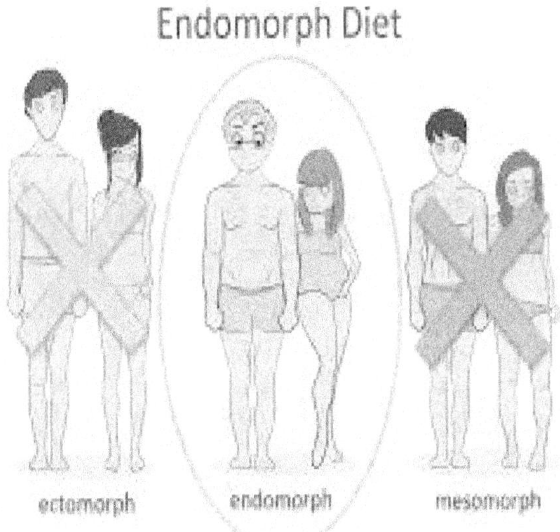

First and foremost, there are 3 totally different kinds of body type, they include the accompanying:

-Endomorphs

-Ectomorphs

-Mesomorphs

a) Endomorphs

This just alludes to the arrangements of people who will in general have a body type that is bigger or bigger, and the rapidly put on weight effortlessly. Furthermore, they likewise fight with their fat levels in their body. Furthermore, this sort of body is regular in the two people, in any case, the ladies society have more difficulties with consuming these overabundance fats.

b) Ectomorphs

It alludes to the class or classifications of individuals that are generally slight and tall, and they discover hard to add weight.

c) Mesomorphs

It basically insinuates individuals that appear to be athletic and strong, notwithstanding a tendency to accommodatingly control or grasp their weight.

Even more thusly, endomorphs react unreasonably quick to extreme use of food sources, by essentially doing a limit of the extra calories as fat right in the variety of such individuals. On the other hand, mesomorphs are good for building muscles without any problem.

Along these lines, if you are an endomorph, and you need to seize your weight similarly as prosperity, you basically need a respectable eating routine game plan notwithstanding the right exercise schedule that be of help to you in a short time.

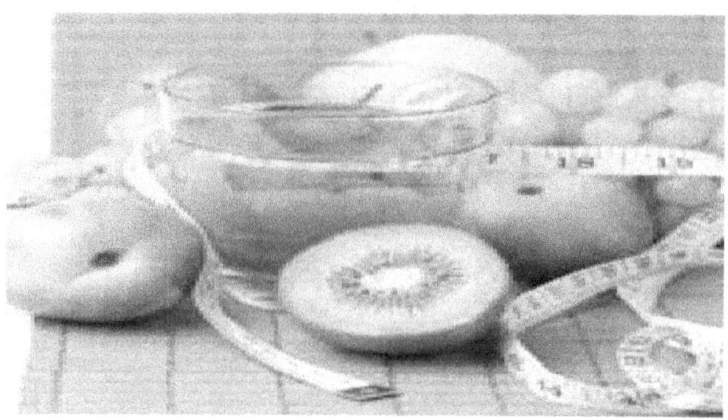

CHAPTER 4

SAMPLE PLAN DIETS & EFFICIENT EXERCISES RECOMMENDED FOR ENDOMORPHS

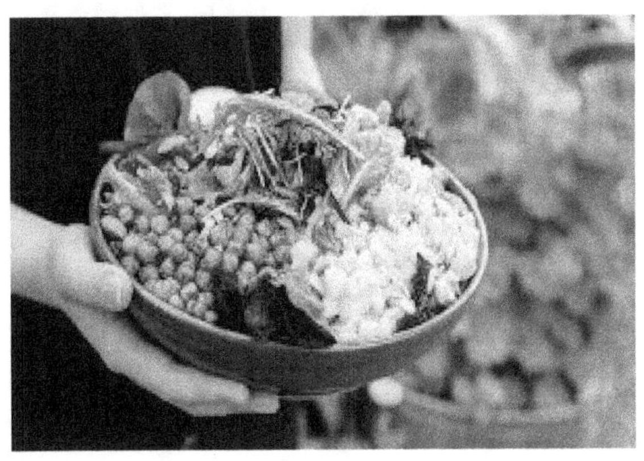

Your arrangement of test feast or diet goes through

your morning meal, lunch as in addition to suppers; just as the indispensable clarifications to these are as per the following:

a) Breakfast

Here, you need shriveled spinach, half avocado, two eggs that are mixed in addition to a touch of chicken frankfurter.

b) Lunch

Here, you need non-starch veggies you like, four ounces of chicken that is heated in addition to a serving of mixed greens various types of greens. Additionally, you need low fat for dressing and without option of sugar. Also, you can make the mixing of the dressing comfortable by basically utilizing balsamic vinegar or maybe olive as the significant fixing.

c) Dinner

Here, you need low fat cheddar, or a hand loaded up with low or diminished salted nuts, one cup of broccoli that is steamed, custom made stew just as normal peanut butter having a touch of full wheat saltines or an apple.

Amazing Endomorph Diet Exercises for You

Presently, endomorph suppers or diets don't just need you taking the indispensable food sources or diets, it additionally expects you to do imperative activities in the proper manners.

Also, if need to consume some fat or get more fit in the correct manner, at that point you essentially need to do a blend of cardiovascular exercise just as strength preparing for a time of four to multiple times consistently; since this training will assist you with managing down or consume 250 calories. Furthermore, to add to the cycle or strategy, cut down your day by day utilization of suppers or food. Also, teach yourself by guaranteeing you complete actual exercise consistently for span of 30 minutes.

Other Necessary Exercises for Endomorphs:

- Dead-lifts

- Pull ups just as jawline ups

- Chest presses

- Squats back and front

- Lunges

- Overhead presses

- Step ups

- Rows

- Dips

CHAPTER 5

THE NECESSARY RULES

The significant notwithstanding specific things you should do or avoid are carefully explained as such:

- Ensure you sit less similarly as move more. for instance you should do walking more

rather than gaze at the TV for
the duration of the day.

- regarding your wellbeing
level, you should be locked in
with strength getting ready
reliably or period; assume 2 to
different occasions in seven
days range, since muscles
improvement will cause you to
lose fat in your body right
away

- Try to know the level of your calories reliably.

- Try whatever amount as could be required to be consistent, and screen your progression by basically taking assessments of your weight for six to multi week stretch as this will engage you to achieve what you significantly need right away.

- consistently, endeavor and drink 80 to 128 ounces of unadulterated water right away

- Consume insignificant notwithstanding visit meals containing sound fats, strong carbs notwithstanding lean protein.

- Ensure you search for the help of a partner or a mentor

that will enable you during the action or cycle.

- For every three to four days time frame, promise you give yourself a cheat diet right away.

- Lastly, attempt however much you can to keep down your pressure; in light of the fact that your feeling of anxiety could affect the whole exercise measure.

THE END

www.ingramcontent.com/pod-product-compliance
Lightning Source LLC
Chambersburg PA
CBHW060923130726

48001CB00006B/2395